The Life and Times of the Baby Catcher

– LIZ BANKS –

An environmentally friendly book printed and bound in
England by www.printondemand-worldwide.com

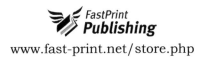

www.fast-print.net/store.php

The Life and Times of the Baby Catcher
Copyright © Liz Banks 2012

ISBN 978-178035-507-8

First published 2012 by
FASTPRINT PUBLISHING
Peterborough, England.
Printed by Printondemand-Worldwide

Acknowledgements

Thanks to family and friends, for your encouragement, you have all helped me at one time or another, some of you by believing in me and some of you by not believing in me. Sometimes a push is as good as a hug but not always.

Starting Out

I left school at 15 with no idea what I wanted to do other than what I had wanted to do from a very young age, become a nurse when I was old enough. I had no idea how to find out about this and it was difficult to get information in those days, the late 1950s

The 'Careers Office' was useless and suggested that I go into office work and sent me for an interview with The Calculating Bureau near to Priory Road in Edgbaston, Birmingham.

I was duly taken on knowing nothing about office work or office machinery, no problem; I was sat at a Power Samas (punch card) machine and shown the rudiments.

The operator had a sheaf of Co-op 'Divi' receipts on the left hand side and the keyboard, operated by the right hand, and spent the working day tapping in the 'divi' number and amount spent. This produced a card with the relevant details in holes and then went to a sorting machine, a verifier, which picked up any mistakes or if there was a bent pin in your machine it would punch the same hole in every card and the whole lot had to be done again and we're talking 2000 cards a hour!!!. BORING.

There were 10 machines in the office, very close together and the noise was terrific, (no ' elf and safety then), and the mindless tapping in of numbers was awful, I dreamed numbers every night for weeks and one of the girls had a nervous breakdown and had to leave.

After I'd been there a while I could shut out the noise and have a conversation at normal level. All of this is now defunct and has been taken over by modern technology. Machines that once filled a whole room are now contained in very small packages. Amazing and wonderful and the things you can do with a smart phone are phenomenal.

At the Calculating Bureau the office boys not only ran the office but another of their duties was to burn the used sanitary towels of the office girls and they'd have a bonfire every couple of days in the field at the back of the office. Yes, a field at the back of the office which was on the main Bristol road into Birmingham!! We also played football in this field at break time; we were all just kids after all.

I was terminally shy (yes me!) there was major embarrassment if anyone spoke to me and fear of speaking to report problems, so problems that could have been avoided became worse and all because I was frightened. Fortunately my supervisor recognised this and was very kind.

The pay was great, I was earning £5 a week and was allowed to keep some for myself but I had to pay my bus fares and dinners out of it. Each Friday lunchtime I would go to Selly Oak village and buy the latest hit records, which included Emile Ford singing 'What do you want to make those eyes at me for?' and Pat Boone, of course, my big favourite. On Thursday evenings we still held the Pat Boone fan club at my house with my school friends, 15 minutes of Pat Boone on Radio Luxemburg, wonderful.

I stayed at The Calculating Bureau for about a year and then saw an advert for a Power Samas operator for Midland Counties Dairy in Birmingham city near to the fire station which was quite a jaunt but the money was better, the office smaller and the work more varied. I was now earning £7 a week, what riches!

Nursing

One of the women in the office (Lily) pointed out an advert in the Evening Mail that said that they were looking for applicants to join the school of nursing in Bromsgrove General Hospital. Nursing was what I had always wanted to do so I wrote and was surprised to get an interview, mum came with me and got on really well with Nora Field, the matron, as mum had been a nurse herself and they were of similar age and were both Scottish.

However matron was not impressed with my attire, as she put it, she thought my heels were too high and not at all sensible. I was wearing a pair of my sister Pats' shoes which were apricot in colour and had 3"stiletto heels and I could hardly walk in them. Pat was really annoyed when she found out as I hadn't asked her if I could borrow them, mainly because I knew she'd say no.

As I had no GCE's (our school didn't do GCE's!) I had to take an entrance exam and did pretty well and so was accepted for general nurse training to start in October which I did, only to be told after 2 weeks that I was, in fact, too young at only 17 ½ and would be employed as an auxiliary nurse student until I was 18 and could legally start my training, which is what happened.

The Hospital

The hospital was an old American army base hospital, as were many in the 50's and 60's, rows of huts joined by a main corridor with gardens in between. It was built behind the old hospital. The original building was built as a poor house and then used as a workhouse and eventually, when the army base was built the front building became administrative offices and the other large building became the geriatric wards. The front building is now grade 2 listed.

The nurses' home was the same design and was run by the home sister who supervised the running of the nurse's home, giving out fresh laundry every week, putting our clean uniforms in our rooms and generally seeing to the smooth running of it all. We all had our own rooms, not big but adequate and comfortable. In fact the first year I was there all the rooms were wallpapered which was a great innovation at the time and made it more homely.

It was my first time away from home, in fact for all of us it was first time away from home. I think we all went a little wild at having what we thought of as our freedom but nothing really bad. Loud music, loud voices and basically loud everything

There was a great mixture of cultures and classes which was great. Maureen was Irish and had never worn knickers before she came to England. Her family used to live in the country and had pheasant for Christmas dinner and pretended it was chicken like the rich people!!!

Aileen was from the West Indies and was older than the rest of us and very homesick,

There were 2 sisters from Ceylon (as it was then) Phyllis was very earnest and did well but her sister, Sonia, was here for a good time and ended up as a cleaner.

My best friends were Barty Barton and Silvia who was known as Lettuce because of her green framed glasses like Lettuce Leaf in the comic, Jenny and I were close friends and there were others, of course Vivienne, Sylvia, Shirley and Gloria (Glossy) springs to mind as she was such a nice person, Penny Coin. I don't remember what her real name was; we called her Penny because of her surname. I was called Liz for the first time in my life and loved it as I was always called Elizabeth at home. We were a fairly tight little group and got on really well together.

There were also male nurses and this was my first encounter with MEN who turned out to be little boys in disguise!! There were psychiatric nurses, seconded to do general nurse training and those doing their general nurse training, about six in all.

In our group there was only one male, Les, a Liverpudlian with a wicked sense of humour and a cruel twist, especially for our wrists. He sat behind me in the classroom and one day, just to make me jump in the middle of a lecture, he stabbed me in the neck with his pen. I shouted, the lecturer stopped and we all looked innocent. No ratting in our camp. Mooney just smiled benignly!

What we wore

First and second year students wore blue and white striped dresses with a full bib apron and blue belt. There was a hat called a butterfly which came from the laundry as a starched oblong and it was really difficult to get the hang of making up but once learned never forgotten, I can still make one now. It was a round top that sat on your head with a pleated tail that hung down at the back.

Once you got to the third year you wore the same dress but had a Sister Dora hat which was more of a square and sat more easily on your head. This hat was very formally presented to you by Matron, you had to kneel at her feet and she put on your hat in the preferred position (preferred by her) over your forehead!! The first thing you did when leaving the office was push it to the back of your head where it felt more comfortable and as far as we were concerned, looked much more cool. We also had a cloak, which I loved, which we wore when it was cold to go from the nurses home to the wards or the school of nursing. These cloaks were black outside with a red lining and cross over straps and were really warm.

Training

Our training began with 3 months in school during which time we learned the basics of anatomy, physiology, nursing care and a lot about the community at large. I remember going to the sewage works which was fascinating and although we were assured that the water that came out at the end of the process was pure neither the man in charge nor any of us was prepared to try it AND he wouldn't let his dog drink it...... Hmmmm

We were also taken to a large block of flats in Birmingham where there was a new system of waste disposal called the Garche system. I've never seen or heard of it since although the masher disposal system in some of the more recent kitchens comes close.

We also had many lectures and sessions in the practical room to prepare us for the rigours of the wards, we learned how to do a bed bath, an enema, an injection (practising with water in a syringe and an orange) and a dry dressing. We also learned the rudiments of laying up a sterile dressing trolley. Nothing too difficult, so far.

After this initial period was over we had a 2 week study block every 3 months and clinical teaching on the wards. We were also assessed at frequent intervals. It sounds quite intense and it was but we learned and there were very few who failed their exams.

In due course we were allocated to the wards. We spent 3 months on each ward and were watched over like babies. At that time we were only allowed to do basic things like cleaning, giving bedpans and bottles for the men and, of course the horror of horrors the metal sputum pots which had to be emptied and cleaned every day, Believe me you only ever dropped one once!!!!

Wards

My first ward was the private ward, ward 10 and the sister was a lovely woman who was so kind to me. The staff nurse on the ward was married and still working at 24 years of age, much to my horror. I was shocked at the time and now here I am still working at 68yrs!!!!!!!!!!!!!!!!!

I don't remember being told the shift times but I'm sure that I was, even so when working a late shift I was sent to tea at 4o'clock and thought that I was finished for the day so didn't go back. The ward sister told me, the next day that my shift actually finished at 8pm. Embarrassing or WHAT?

We worked a 48 hour week, the shifts were

7.30 – 10 and then 2 – 8pm.

7.30 – 1 and then 5 – 8pm

7.30 – 5pm

Night duty was 8 – 8am

When I was on nights for the first time, I was working on ward 10 alone but with someone on call. There were only 2 patients and as I was cold in the middle of the night I sat in the office with my nice warm cloak around me. I don't know how long I was there but was suddenly aware of the night sister standing in front of me. He said not to be alarmed as I had night nurse paralysis which would go away very quickly and to call him when I was OK, also that my patients were sleeping and safe.

I have never forgotten the awful feeling of not being able to move and how kind Mr Whitehead was, he was right, it passed quickly and has never happened to me again.

I enjoyed my time on ward 10 and learned a lot, mostly hospital politics! Specialling a patient, involved sitting with a post-op patient until he came around from the anaesthetic. Later in our training we were to be given much more intense one to one patient care.

I remember making boiled egg and mayonnaise sandwiches for the private patients' tea and eating most of the filling!!

The matron caught my friend and I one day in the kitchen and bade us good day, as I had a mouthful of dry Horlicks powder at the time I couldn't answer but she demanded that I minded my manners so I did and she was sprayed with said powder at which she huffed and walked out, phew!

Matron could be a dragon but was also fair in her dealings. We were told don't stand if you can sit, don't sit if you can lie but heaven help you if you're caught!

Staff meals were served in the dining room and everyone had their place, students on the left hand tables and staff nurses on the right, senior nurses in the middle. Sometimes matron helped serve the meals and everyone ate in silence when she was there AND ate everything that she put on your plate!!!!! Choice, what choice?

If she walked through the dining room everyone stood to attention until she left. Everyone took this for granted as simply good manners.

I remember in the classroom when we were asked what to do if we met matron in the corridor and one of the girls suggested that we curtsey, of course the right answer was only speak if spoken to otherwise just keep going.

Other rules that applied to matron were that if you were summoned to her office then you rushed back to your room and put on a clean apron and combed your hair. In the office you always stood in front of matrons' desk with hands behind your back and waited to be spoken to.

Christmas

On the wards there had to be complete silence with all patients in their beds, looking tidy, when the consultants did their rounds, all very solemn. If a consultant came onto the ward, in fact if anyone senior to you came onto the ward you were expected to stand up and speak only when spoken to.

On Christmas day everyone worked but we were all given time to visit the other wards and admire both the decorations, the food and the alcohol, everyone ended up a little tipsy, including matron and the assistant matrons. Imagine that happening now. HUH!

Every ward had a turkey and one of the consultants was there to carve and serve dinner to staff and patients.

As many patients as possible were sent home so it was usually quiet and as we didn't have a casualty department we didn't have emergencies very often.

Christmas also meant the Matrons Ball, a grand affair with everyone in evening dress, a live band and good food and drink but no-one got drunk......... It was usually held in the ballroom of the local psychiatric hospital and the patients that were able to be, were included.

It was really quite strange and a little frightening as we had to be escorted, all of us in evening dress, from the front door of the hospital to the ballroom with a porter with a huge bunch of keys to open doors and lock them behind us.

It's very sad to say that most of these places have now disappeared. There were a lot of the old psychiatric hospitals that were set in large grounds, many of them had their own farms which were worked by the able bodied patients and were self-sufficient. All gone. Now the able bodied are in the community and care is hard to find.

Also we didn't suffer from racism or political correctness at the time; people were judged on their attitude, ability and friendliness.

Wards: - 11 Male medical

There was an old man who tried to escape from the men's medical. He was a very small man who wanted to go home in the middle of a very cold night; he had dementia and was quite violent in his confusion. It took four of us to restrain him and a fifth to inject him with a drug called Paraldehyde which was effective but smelled like tomcat wee, horrible and the patient smelled of it for days afterwards as it was excreted via urine, faeces, breath and sweat. He was eventually transferred to the geriatric ward as he had no family and could never cope on his own. Very sad.

Then there was a confused old man when I was on night duty that trapped me under the cot he was in. What happened was that one side of the cot was down and I had gone to the other side to pick up something he had dropped under the bed and he dropped the other side on me. I was really embarrassed as I had to wait for my colleague to come back from her dinner break to let me out.

I remember smoking Park Drive cigarettes with him to stop him shouting in the middle of the night and waking everyone else in the ward. Those Park Drive were really strong.

One day the ward sister asked him what she should do with me and his reply –'you should always look for the good and I´m sure the good will overcome the bad'. I don't think she was convinced.

Sister really didn't like male nurses and Keith Jones, a male student nurse, was so frustrated by her that he threw a bucket of water on the floor in front of her one day and marched off. When asked why, he told her that it was better on the floor than on her head. She was speechless and then let a little smile through. Or it could have been wind!! (Old midwives joke!)

And then there was Dizzy Mary, an older staff nurse who went around the patients each day with her 'bowel book', she also carried, with her, the suppository tray, just in case!! Surprising how many patients were 'asleep' when she came into view!

One thing that was NOT allowed on the ward was a bedsore as it suggested that we were not doing our job properly and also invited the wrath of matron who gave us a real dressing down when a patient was admitted with one.

With our good care they healed fairly quickly. Thank heavens.

Ward 12 - Female Medical Ward

Sister Brennan – so young to be a sister, I was amazed at her being a sister when she was only in her 20's. She was sooo kind to me, in fact, to everyone.

On that ward there was an old lady who painted the toilet walls and the toilet itself with poo, and her hands as well but as she told us, she was just helping it out!

Ward cleaning. First job in the morning, while the patients had their breakfast we made the beds and had the report and after breakfasts were cleared away the junior nurses and auxiliaries did the ward cleaning. All the beds were pulled away from the wall and every surface cleaned with a damp cloth. Coffee or tea was served at 10.30 and all patients were given drinks and we ensured that they drank them. Meal times on the ward were the same and even though feeding patients who were not capable of feeding themselves was an onerous task, it was accepted as part of nursing care.

Ward 8 - Gynaecology

I didn't know that I was expected to listen to the report and remember what was said!! There were so many patients that I couldn't believe that we were expected to remember them all. Time and practice and seeing patients as people proved that it was possible!

Pubic shaves were done for almost everything, from D and Cs' to hysterectomies and all patients were given a wash, (a vulval toilet) and put into a clean nightie on their return from theatre. Nursing care as it should be.

The ward sister didn't like me and was very impatient which made me even more nervous but it ended up being my favourite ward.

Ward 9 - Paediatrics

Children I remember include David the 5 year old boy that drowned, he was at the pub by the canal with his parents and friends, he disappeared and when they finally found him under the dock he was resuscitated and spent many weeks hanging on to life before he finally died. What a tragedy. Then there were the children that were gassed, in a suicide attempt by their mother. They also succumbed.

My nephew, Stephen vomited copious amounts of red 'stuff' after his eye operation which frightened the nurse looking after him as she thought it was blood, actually it was undiluted Ribena to which he had helped himself from the bottle.

Ward 5 - Female Surgery

My introduction to doing dressings was almost mystical, I felt like a real nurse at last as I was instructed on the laying up of trolleys. The ritual of disinfecting, sterilizing and laying out of the sterile dressings and covering them with a sterile towel all done with long handled forceps called Cheatles, not an easy task. The dressing itself was a bit of anti-climax as it was just a cover over an appendix scar.

First colostomy!!!!!! A colostomy is when a part of the bowel and rectum is removed and the cut end is opened onto the tummy wall and a bag catches the stools. Oh! That first colostomy. The smell and trying to ignore it for the patients' sake. The terrible sore area around the wound and the awful sticky on the bags that repeatedly took off some of the skin making it worse. Thank God, that such strides have been made in post op colostomy care.

Shaving pre-op patients was always the last job of the shift and you could almost guarantee a veritable ape who took ages to shave and always meant that you were late off duty, usually when your social life was waiting.

During our time on the wards we were all teased and tricked into things like go to theatre and ask for a long stand, (the person in charge would say OK and tell you to wait, then come along 10 minutes later and tell you could go back now, your stand was long enough) or to ward 8 to ask for a left handed fallopian tube, everyone played along and we soon learned which were real and which were not. One trick that was used on new students was the urine tasting trick. They were shown how to test the urine by putting a finger in the specimen and then tasting it to see if there was sugar in it, of course the finger that was put in the urine was NOT the finger that you put in your mouth but they didn't notice that!!! A bit mean but quite funny to watch.

Physiotherapy dept.

Was where we played table tennis in the evenings, the whole department, even the whole hospital was riddled with cockroaches and as we opened the door and turned on the lights we would hear them running for cover and see a black tide widening like the rolling back of the Red Sea. I still hate cockroaches and have never found a use for them.

We also used the physiotherapy department for the Christmas production each year. These consisted of skits, songs, dances and recitals. The senior staff were lampooned and took it all in good part and a good time was had by all. I still have the picture of myself and 5 others doing the Can Can.

Naughty Nurses, innocent style.

The night we put Keith's' room out on the grass, we were always up to mischief and one night put all the furniture from Keith's room out on the grass between the blocks of the nurses home. As he walked past on his way to his room he laughed and said that some poor bugger was in for a surprise, he was NOT amused when he found it was his room however and he knew immediately that I was involved as I had written on his mirror, in toothpaste, POOR KIETH. I could never remember how to spell his name.

Creeping in after lights out. We were expected to be in our rooms by 10 o'clock, matron took her role of loco parentis very seriously. Sometimes we were, sometimes we weren't. The night sister would come around every block and call lights out and we would, of course comply!! As I say, sometimes we were there and sometimes we weren't and sometimes we would all be together in one room waiting for night sister to leave before we put the lights and the music back on but more quietly and carry on partying. I'm sure they knew but said nothing.

In the morning it was the night sister who woke us up by banging on each bedroom door with a spoon and even if you had a sign saying DAY OFF you still heard all the other doors being banged.

Ward 16

Ward 16 was the pub over the road called The Hop Pole.

Bromsgrove was a quiet little town, the most exciting things there were the cinema, the coffee bar and the pubs but we didn't go into the pubs much. It was so quiet that returning from a 'night out' we could, and did, lie in the middle of the main road and wait for a car to come. Most times it was a long wait or we gave up. That road is very busy both day and night now so no more lying around!!!!

I was the first one at the hospital to have a mini dress (only about 2 inches above the knee but quite shocking at the time). I loved that dress and wore it until it almost fell to bits. Matron wasn't impressed as she told me, 'Nurse Earle, I can see your popliteal space!!'

This is the space behind your knee, shock horror!

David driving the mini down the main corridor but this was much later and I was already working in London and only back for a visit.

Geriatrics

One Christmas I was allocated to the geriatric wards and wasn't overly pleased but the four of us who were allocated made the best of it and treated the patients well, which is more than can be said for some of the permanent staff! Especially an SEN on night duty who used to beat the men with his walking stick, no-one saw him do it but the bruises were there and they were all frightened of him. Mistreatment of the elderly is not new it's always been there. This one was known as John the limp. He was one of the few assistant nurses that were given their State Enrolled Nurse status in the 1950s, for long service but no formal training a terrible thing to do but fortunately it died out and the ones who were left were almost at retiring age then.

We decorated the ward for Christmas and the patients wept as they had not had decorations before. Such a simple thing to give so much pleasure. It made me feel ashamed that no-one else had bothered.

Geriatrics that I remember clearly are – Mary who sang Daisy, Daisy (give me your answer do), in such a frail little voice, she used to lie curled up in her bed like a little dormouse.

The woman next to her who said that she had a big black African worm inside her, this along with her tales of the dirty woman who slept with her lodger who was a black man, led to much speculation!!

There was a woman who was admitted while I was there who sat in her place in the day room and looked out of the window saying over and over 'I wish I was a dickie bird, I'd fly away from here'.

And then there was the patient who gave us 'sweeties' wrapped in newspaper, except they weren't sweeties they were lumps of poo. You were only ever caught out once and thereafter just said thank you and put them in the bin.

One day there was a fight in the men's dayroom. Two men who sat opposite each other had an argument, as neither could walk they simply threw themselves towards each other as far as they could and were lying on the floor, lashing out at each other with their walking sticks. What pandemonium.

Then there was the incident of the sanichair which brought tears to the eyes. A sanichair is like a wheelchair but it has a toilet seat that you can wheel your patient over the toilet but you had to ensure that when you went to take a male patient out of the toilet that he had raised his undercarriage.

Sadly one day I was in a hurry and pulled the chair to his screams of BACK UP! BACK UP! No permanent damage was done but apologies were profuse.

Although we hadn't been keen to work on the geriatric wards, we learned a lot about nursing care, about talking to people, about appreciating their lives, about ourselves and about people in general.

Theatre

I hated theatre. I hated scrubbing up and I hated cleaning. Every morning we would clean the theatre and anaesthetic rooms using a wet cloth we would wash up as far as we could reach and down to the floor, all walls and equipment included.

The only thing good about theatre was the doctor that I was seeing at the time who protected me from the wrath of the theatre sister who had her favourites (not me!!!) including the surgeon who brought his dog into the main theatre, to spay her. He was even still wearing his muddy wellies!!

One day, when it was my turn to scrub, the patient was a lady with varicose veins in both legs which were to be stripped. Theatre was running a bit late and it was decided that it would be a good idea to have a surgeon on each leg at the same time to do a bilateral varicose vein stripping, with me and the instrument trolley in between, it worked well for me as, eventually I just stood back and let them help themselves to the instruments and it worked well for them as they got the right instruments as they needed them!!!!

I just kept the trolley tidy and the needles ready in their holders.

Years later I learned to love theatre as we had our own obstetric theatre in Redditch and were expected to scrub if there was a caesarean section or in an emergency.

Seconded

As we had no casualty department at Bromsgrove we were sent to Kidderminster hospital to do our casualty training. We had a great time; the work was fascinating, exciting and horrifying at times.

The carpet factories were centred in Kidderminster at that time and I remember a young man coming into casualty having caught his hands in the carpet rollers and both were completely degloved, poor man, he was rapidly shipped off to another hospital which specialised in such injuries and we never did hear what happened to him.

We stayed in the nurse's home and as at Bromsgrove we were expected to be in by 10pm. Fat chance!! I'd still like to know who it was who put the toilet cleaner tins back on the window sill every time that I had so carefully moved so that we could get back in through the toilet window without making a noise. Still, we rarely got caught. After 3 months we were glad to get back to our wider circle of friends having completed all of the skills that were required of us in casualty.

Seniority

Last man in was bottom of the pile and if someone was even just 3 months ahead of you they were your seniors and you did as they said. Well, most of the time. Cold baths were the initiation, fully dressed of course.

This included new doctors as long as they were friendly. There was a gorgeous looking new chap that we all ogled, he was so friendly and pleasant and wore purple suede shoes, just right for dunking!! Boy was he mad as his shoes were completely ruined and his feet were purple.

During this time we had girlfriends and boyfriends outside of the hospital but it was rare to have relationships other than friendship within the groups.

Having completed my general nurse training I was sorry to leave Bromsgrove hospital which had been so good for me allowing me to grow up in safety and friendship without ever realizing that was what was happening.

I feel that the students of today have gained much in their freedom but lost out on all the fun that we had.

From Bromsgrove I moved to -

Bishops Stortford Hospital, Essex

This was a small, cosy general hospital, where they did minor surgery it was run on ancient lines, where the staff were spoon fed cod liver oil and malt every morning by the ward sister!

On the children's ward there was a little boy who escaped. He was 5 years old and was due to have a circumcision the next day and was very frightened as he thought we were going to cut off his 'willy'. I had been down the ward and seen him go to the toilet and he was OK. Less than half an hour later there was a phone call from his parents to ask how he was, and I told them that he was fine. They then told me that they already knew this as he was in his bed at home. Apparently when he went to the toilet he had climbed out of the window and taken himself home.... Over the main road and over the level crossing!!!!!!!!! He never did have his circumcision.

Then there was the student nurse who was on secondment from another hospital who I had asked to wash and remake the bed of a patient who had been discharged. When I went to look for her sometime later I found the curtains pulled around and her asleep on the bed and having woken her was treated to a tirade of curses. She told me that in her country she was a princess and she would have the witch doctor put a spell on me. I asked could she possibly wash and make up the bed before doing this and left her to it. The next thing I knew was that she had reported me to the matron for waking her up. Matron wasn't impressed and the girl was sent back to her training hospital very soon after that.

Bishops Stortford was a very quiet little town but it had 2 advantages, one was the American Air base that had regular dances and not only invited the hospital staff but also collected us and brought us back. We had such a lot of laughs with these men and were so well looked after. I was seeing a chap called Groucho (because he looked like Groucho Marx, complete with moustache.) and renamed myself Angelique, he called me Angel, of course, bless him, always the perfect gentleman. I lost a shoe one evening and he carried me down the drive to where the bus was waiting to take us home. I was only about 8 stone then so his back was safe! How things change. I don't think that he'd manage to carry me now!!

The second advantage was the London fire brigade training school which also had social nights which were not so well behaved and VERY social but that's a story for another time.

There was also a third advantage in that my sister Jo and her family lived not too far away and I could visit them on my days off, which was great and kept me steady, well, steadyish.

Janet, my friend and partner in crime (such as it was, involving only having a good time when off duty) had a family with a history of cancer her brother had cancer of the kidney, her mother had breast cancer, Janet had breast cancer and even the dog had breast cancer. What a tragedy, such a lovely family. Life is cruel at times. I used to stay with them when Janet and I had the same days off and one time I had to do CPR on the mother when she had a heart attack and managed to bring her back before the ambulance came.

Bishops Stortford was a very happy place for me and it allowed me to spend time with my sister Jo and her family but there was very little chance of advancement so I moved to -

Princess Elizabeth in Harlow

Where I went to start my midwifery training but I wasn't ready for the studying at that time. I was much entangled with my love life and life in general so only lasted 3 months and then went back to Birmingham and stayed with Mum for a while before getting a job at the North Middlesex hospital in London.

There were a few memorable things about Harlow, one is the time that I was in the antenatal clinic with the consultant who wanted to examine the woman he was with so I set her up on the examination couch to be greeted with loud laughter, the poor woman had gone to the toilet prior to this and having wiped herself with a tissue from her pocket and had left a green shield stamp stuck to her pubic hair. 'Hmmmm,' said the consultant,' we're being given Green Shield Stamps, now!'

Harlow was where I saw the biggest new born baby I have ever seen he was 13pounds and looked about 3 months old. A normal delivery, both of his parents were large folk but even so, it made my eyes water!

My next move was to -

North Middlesex Hospital

I moved to London next and worked for a time as a staff nurse on night duty and was then offered a post as night sister, a great honour as I was the youngest night sister they had ever had and the apple of the matrons eye until I became pregnant but more of that later.

I have always found it easy to make friends and been very lucky to have had so many good friends. The North Mid was no exception and life was very good. Work was a never ending round of 'occurrences' like the night I was called to the male orthopaedic ward by an hysterical staff nurse because he couldn't control the young men in his ward who had balled up sheets of newspaper and thrown them into the middle of the ward and were now throwing lighted matches at it, little devils, they made that poor guys life a real trial. I confiscated all matches, read them the riot act put the lights out and left. Job done!!

When it was quiet we spent a fair bit of time in the switch board, keeping the switchboard operator company. One night we were messing about and rang the mortuary for a laugh and nearly died of fright when the phone was answered. It was a Rabbi who was sitting with a man that had died that day.

The medical block at the North Mid was out in the grounds which were very dark at night and I dreaded being allocated there. One night as I was crossing the gardens for the middle round, about 2 o'clock, I saw a man jump out of a second floor window and run off across the grounds. It turned out to be a Mr Liquorish who had wanted to go home. We called the police and a search was made but he was never heard from again.

A number of times, as I raced over the gardens to get to the safety of the wards in the dead of night, I dropped my bleep or whatever I was carrying and had to go back for them, aaagggghhhhhhh!! There were lots of trees and big shrubs in those gardens and it was scary in the dark.

There was a particularly scary corridor going out to the psychiatric unit where I went to visit Trevor who was a night sister there but I was always very wary as he had some quite violent patients and it wasn't a locked ward. There was Big John and the threat of violence. I have never come across such, dare I say evil, in a man's eyes as John who came striding through the office door one night as we were having coffee, shouting and banging about, Trevor was very calm and coped with it all wonderfully but it could have been nasty. I was very pregnant at the time too and was very frightened by the incident.

After I had been at the North Mid for a while living in the nurses home, I moved into a flat with a girl called Wendy who had had a baby when she was 15 years old and her parents had made her give it up for adoption which Wendy had never got over. Despite her sadness she was a good flatmate. The flat was in a place called Angel Place and was fine but very small, we later moved to a bigger place in Tottenham, just behind the football ground, very noisy on Saturdays but a friendly place to live. Great party on cup final day 1967!!

Wendy eventually moved on and I was invited to share a flat with 2 friends who had a little boy, they lived in Wood Green and were happy to have another person to share the rent and childcare as by that time I was pregnant, and it worked very well. I had met David at a party whilst I was visiting my sister in Birmingham over the Christmas holiday, he came down to see me a few times especially when Liverpool was playing, hence cup final day!!

The party on cup final day proved to be very productive it was when I became pregnant!!!!!!!!!

I knew that I had to tell matron and it was whilst handing over the night report one morning that she told me about a 'silly girl' on the staff that was pregnant AGAIN. To which I replied, so am I. She was totally shocked and asked when I was getting married to which I replied that I wasn't.

It was at this point that I became her 'unfavourite' and was told that I could work until I was 28 weeks pregnant and after that she did not wish to see me again. Maternity leave was only for married staff but the law said that women could work until they reached twenty eight weeks of their pregnancy. Now women can work right up until they go into labour as long as she and the baby are well. Sometimes I think that this is a good thing and sometimes not.

Such was the power of the matron that she could make me leave at twenty eight weeks and refuse to have me back... I contacted all sorts of people to try and change this but couldn't, her word was law. I think that the best thing that came from that meeting with matron was that from then on we were allowed to sit down to give and receive the report as, if I had to stand, I fainted and they had to interrupt the report to haul me off to a chair .

Every cloud has a silver lining!!!

Unmarried mothers were definitely frowned upon in 1968 despite what you hear about the swinging 60's and life could have been very hard for me but I had a great deal of support through my pregnancy and I was really healthy except for the anaemia that was brought on by my vast consumption of Rennies which I didn't need but I just had to have them, I ended up having to have injections of iron and was left with brown stains on my bum for about 18 months. My other cravings were for golden delicious apples and lager, how wicked AND I smoked.

I told David, well, actually I didn't tell him. What happened was that he was living in the midlands and I went up to see my family when I was about 6 months pregnant and he asked me to go for a drink with him, I said yes and he picked me up, when we got to the pub he helped me off with my coat and sat down in shock. His first words were 'bloody hell, I'd get drunk if I could afford it'. And his next words were 'When do you want to get married?' Being an independent sort of person I said that I didn't and so we kept in touch by post.

Motherhood

My son was born in March 1968 and from the beginning he was not a happy baby, he cried endlessly and to try to satisfy him I fed him far too much which made things worse. Being a nurse doesn't automatically endow you with wisdom where your own children are concerned!!

The stress of living with an unhappy baby whilst sharing a flat and trying to work and trying to get some sleep was awful but my friends were so good and helped all they could. Their little boy of 4 years loved Marc and would sit with him and sing.

Marc was christened at 6 weeks and we had a party with lots of people including David who got a little boisterous and pushed a daffodil into my ear, strange the things you remember.

As I was not welcome back at the North Middlesex hospital I worked for an agency which meant that I could arrange my work to fit in with my friends to cover child care for our children. It was exhausting but needs must....

On a positive note, I worked at lots of different places and learned a lot. Some of the places that I worked –

The Middlesex Hospital

I worked on the recovery ward looking after patients who had had brain surgery. Intensive care for sure and very exacting.

Moorefield's eye hospital

Here I had a post op patient jump out of the bathroom window four floors up and kill himself. The surgeon had removed his bandages but as we couldn't find an interpreter to tell him that his sight would improve over a matter of days after his bandages came off, he thought that the operation had failed ad quietly went and committed suicide, what a tragedy.

Another patient tried to teach me a little Chinese but I couldn't get the hang of it, all those nasal noises.

It was generally a pleasant place to work.

There was a convalescent home on Hampstead Heath

This was a wonderful old house where the patients were mostly self-caring and I was only there in case of emergency and to give out any tablets that were required.

The grounds were beautiful and the wildlife fascinating. BUT before I had been given this placement I had had dreams about a green tiled corridor that I was walking along and was terrified because I knew that there was something awful around the corner. Imagine my distress when I went exploring in the middle of the night and found myself in this same corridor. I ran upstairs and shut myself in the office until morning and never went back there again.

And then there was a hospital where a very kind male staff nurse tried to save me from eternal damnation for being an unmarried mother. He tried very hard to convert me to his religion but failed. Sweet man.

Moving Again

It was during this time that my friends decided to move back to the USA and I moved in with my two gay friends Trevor and Tony, lovely guys who were prone to looking after strays. My family was shocked and my mother more than anyone else, I had to explain the difference between gays and paedophiles but she was still not happy. This was beside the point, really because when I had written to her to tell her that I was pregnant she hadn't replied for three months and when she did it was to tell me that I had made my bed and should lie on it !!

Anyway it worked very well with Trevor and Tony, I had all the advantages of male company and protection with no strings attached, they even vetted people that I went out with; they were great with Marc and generally spoilt him rotten. They also had two dogs, Penny and Sally, who would wreck the flat when left on their own and when left shut in the kitchen while we were out they would raid the fridge but only eat the good stuff, like the steak intended for our tea. The funniest time though was when they found a bag of flour and we came home to two white dogs that, at least had the manners to look shamefaced!

When Tony and Trevor decided that they were going to live in Bristol they assumed that I would be going with them which is what happened. We rented a house in Fishponds that I really feel was haunted and it wasn't until a few years later that I found out that the boys felt the same way. The house belonged to an old spinster who had gone on a world cruise. That house didn't like us and was very creepy. I spent a lot of time in the garden that summer.

I hated the house; I hated Fishponds and hated living in Bristol.

Obviously I had to work but until I found a job I applied for unemployment benefits and a social services man duly visited the house and took the necessary information, he also tried to take advantage of my situation by trying to get me to agree with the idea of spending time with him in his caravan at the seaside!!!!!

Strangely enough I declined and never did get any benefits and soon after found a job at a geriatric hospital and worked part time on night duty.

Manor Park hospital

Was an old hospital with historic connections with the slave trade and had been an asylum many years ago, for social misfits, this included young girls from the earlier part of the 20th century that became pregnant and were institutionalised so that the family were spared the shame of unwed motherhood.

There were people who had been born there (the children of these unfortunates), who had grown up in the wards and were taken care of by the patients and never went out. These people occupied a part of the outer block of wards and the staff never went in there which I didn't find out until I did a ward round one night which was really scary as they all just stood and stared at me and didn't say a word. The upstairs staff were amazed that I'd been brave enough to go in there and I never went again. Spooky !!

Bristol lasted about 6 months and then Tony had an accident which led to the boys splitting up and so we all moved again but in different directions. Trevor, to South Africa to the famous Groot Schoor Hospital. Tony, back to London and Marc and myself to another part of London.

I found a job as a house keeper to a Jewish family in central London but this didn't work. I was expected to put my son (who was a very poor sleeper) to bed at 6pm and then spend the evening upstairs with the boss' kids with my son at 2 years of age on his own 6 floors down in a locked room. NO WAY.

I had no idea about Jewish feasts, religious tenets or how to cook. Indeed, I had no idea how to be a housekeeper!! I, sadly, made mistakes that offended them which included doing my washing on a Friday and dropping a large lump of gefilte fish (which spread all over the kitchen floor) but I **was** shown how to skin an ox tongue which was really useful, NOT. They were very kind but it just never would have worked and I left after two weeks.

From there I went to stay at Trevor's parents but this was not ideal as they were not used to children especially not a young child who cried a lot. They were kind but again, it didn't work but I then found a job in a residential nursery where I could have Marc with me full time which suited us both.

Considering the life and times it was surprisingly difficult to find a job that accommodated a single mother and her child. Eventually I found a job at a residential nursery in north London.

Mill hill Nursery

A well run residential council nursery. That had room for about thirty children from birth up to the age of five years.

They were divided into four rooms, different colours; six children in each, ranging from 18months to 5 years, Babies were in a separate wing. Each room had its own nursery nurse who was in charge and an assistant; the children were really well cared for both physically and emotionally. Everything was colour coded, the children all had their own clothes and each room had its own colour coded... everything from plates to curtains.

In the evenings when we were not on call we were free to do as we wished, we would watch TV in the staff lounge (The original Star Trek) or play cards and one evening we had a go at the Ouija board, never again, we frightened ourselves silly and all slept in one room that night. Really grown up!!

I met Connie and her son Gary at the nursery, she was another unwed mum and we hit it off straight away. During my time at the nursery I went back to visit the people that lived in Wood Green, there was the German couple who had an escape artist three year old who drove his mother to distraction at times, so much so that one day she tied him by one leg to the tree in the garden! At other times the cry would go out 'Thomas is gone' and we'd all go in predetermined directions to look for him. One day Thomas was found in the local police station, the only information he would give them was that his name was Thomas the Tank engine.

The couple in the ground floor flat were John and Rose who had a son and a baby daughter, they were what would be described as 'rough diamonds', they'd do anything for you but lived in squalor. You had to be careful where you sat and you NEVER accepted a drink!

Amongst the children that I met in the nursery were, Eddie the escape artist, who needed a net over his cot to stop him from running away at night. Even so he was once found up on the roof! Eddie was three years old and His sister, Monica was five, when Monica was taken out she invariably made a scene and would kick and scream to get attention wherever and whenever she felt the need, in the shops, on the street, in the park, anywhere. She was very difficult to deal with but could also be very loving. I wonder what happened to these children. They were always very happy to come back to the nursery after a visit with their father and there was some hint of abuse whilst they were with him and the visits stopped and the children settled down.

Then there was Melanie, a beautiful little girl with a difficult past, who was adopted twice and returned twice as she was so difficult and the adoptive parents couldn't cope with her. There are a surprising number of adopted children that are returned for one reason or another, even today.

There were some very sad stories to tell about these children and it was no wonder that they were traumatised.

Our next move was to Birmingham. So many moves....

Birmingham Ear Nose and Throat Hospital

I had never done ENT (ear, nose and throat) nursing before, except for looking after children who had had tonsils and adenoids removed. There was such a lot to learn and I learned fast. I was initially employed as a staff nurse and graduated to ward sister. I attended the ENT course at the Queen Elizabeth Hospital in Birmingham and found it fascinating and not a little frightening!

As a staff nurse I worked on the post op ward and also in the recovery room where we would sing to patients as they woke up, one man was convinced that we were angels and that he'd died and gone to heaven. He took some convincing that he was still alive and even recovering, despite the fact that our singing wasn't very tuneful!!

There was some amazing surgery performed at that hospital and the nursing care and after care were second to none but this is another hospital that has, sadly, now gone.

Marc and I initially moved in with Mum and Harry (my stepfather) for a while and then found a flat nearby. Mum looked after Marc until he went to the local nursery and then when he went to school she had him at home time until I finished work.

At that time I had a blond wig, Marilyn Monroe type, that I wore when I had a bad hair day, I was convinced that no-one noticed!!!!!! We can fool ourselves into anything, can't we? No-one ever mentioned it at the time but years later I worked with one of the nursery nurses who had looked after Marc in Birmingham and she told me that I was 'the hoot of the day' when I wore my wig. Let's face it; no-one would ever confuse me with Marilyn Monroe!!!!!!!

One day whilst on the way to drop Marc off at the nursery I went to cross a side road in front of a car that was waiting to pull out of the side road onto the main road, Marc was in the pushchair and as I stepped off the pavement the car pulled away taking us with him, he hadn't looked and so when he hit us he was totally shocked as was I (Marc wasn't bothered!) anyway all was well and we carried on to nursery and work as usual. I thought nothing of this incident until I told a friend a work and she was so shocked at the possibilities.

Marc wasn't happy at nursery and one day ended up in hospital after having a fall so Mum looked after him and they had a great time. They had picnics in the local park, in January!!!! They collected stones from the garden and carried them in a bag for Marc to throw them in the canal, not necessarily educational but great fun.

At this time I resumed my relationship with David which made both Marc and I very happy, we found a flat and moved in together and three weeks later we got married. Connie and Gary came to the wedding, as did Tony, it was lovely to see them again but sadly it was the last time I saw any of them.

We were very happy in that flat, it was light and airy and, OK so all of our furniture was second hand but we did have a new cooker and fridge. The armchairs were from a hairdressers shop and were very upright and even our bed came from a second hand shop.

One of the things that I bought was a bookshelf for Marc's room which I painted in red gloss paint, it looked great and he loved it. Early the next morning we heard him in the bathroom running water and asked what he was doing, to which he replied that he 'couldn't get this paint off mine hands'. At the word paint we both leapt out of bed to find that he'd painted the fridge and the cooker and a cupboard door in red gloss. He told us that he was helping us!!!!!!! We were so busy trying to remove the paint that we forgot to scold him and he was very quiet for the rest of the day and didn't pick up a paint brush for many years.

From the flat we managed to get on the property ladder and bought an old villa style house for £6000 pounds, a huge amount that frightened us to death! It was a sturdy house but freezing in the winter. It was here that we had our third child, Dolly, the dog who never considered herself to be anything other than one of the children.

Selly Oak Hospital

After we were married I moved to Selly Oak hospital on night duty as it worked better with the family, it meant that either David or I were with Marc and was much better all round. I worked Wednesday, Friday and Saturday nights but had to stay up all day Thursday which was very hard but it worked well and lasted for a long time, almost ten years, it was easier after the children went to school as I could grab a few hours' sleep on Thursdays,

I worked as a staff nurse at first and then as a night sister when I went back to work after having our second child, Robert. Marc was four at the time and my life was busy, to say the least!

At night the hospital was divided into 'blocks' for allocation to the night sisters.

These were a mixed bag of specialities comprising at least four wards each. The surgical block included gynaecology, ophthalmology (eyes), ENT and obstetrics. The garden included paediatrics, medical and geriatric wards and the other two were surgical, Genito-urinary and Accident & Emergency.

I mainly covered the surgical block or one of the two medical blocks. Paediatrics, Accident &Emergency, gynaecology and eyes were included as well. If I was covering the garden block it was two medical wards and the paediatrics and the geriatric wards although we didn't do much for them except call in to be sociable and to collect their night reports to hand over to the day staff.

We had many interesting nights especially when a cardiac arrest was called out on the garden block and we were in the office in the main building and all had to run like mad things to get there in time, we did actually save lives despite being unable to breathe after running to get there.

Moving House Again

In 1982 the Bankses (us) moved to Droitwich, to a brand new four bedroom house. Marc was eleven and Rob was seven years old. It was a busy time for me, between running a home, rearing two children and chauffeuring them around to their various activities and working but David helped and we were happy. We all loved the new house and were lucky that all our neighbours had children much the same ages as ours and we all got on well.

When we first moved in the roads weren't built up and all of us would sit on the kerb and chat, sometimes even with a can of beer in hand but only the adults!! The kids had a whale of a time with all the builders 'stuff' that was left lying around, especially the big cable reels which they'd ride up and down the road. Health and Safety? What health and safety?

During this time I decided to do some studying at night school and did GCSE English the first year and the second year English Literature and managed to do well in both. I also derived a great deal of pleasure doing them. I was the oldest on the course!

Over the years I had never lost my wish to do midwifery and my chance came when Worcester Hospital announced that they were going to start the 18 month midwifery course. As the boys were eight and twelve years and were now able to cope with me working full time I grasped the nettle and applied and to my delight got a place on the first group.

Midwifery

There were 12 of us on the course and we were ranged from newly qualified (around 21 years) to middle aged and yet we gelled well as a group. I was, of course the oldest. One of the girls, Heather, had a van and this was made good use of for various trips. One of the trips was to the same sewage works that I had been to as a student nurse 20 years before. No change there and this man wouldn't let his dog drink the end water either. What a laugh.

Midwifery has a totally different culture to general nursing where everyone was addressed by their title or status. In midwifery we were called by our Christian names (except for sister and the upper echelons). Although it took a bit of getting used to, I loved it all and although most of our women were healthy and had healthy babies there was also the possibility of problems arising and having done my general nurse training was definitely an advantage.

I found it challenging, wonderful, frightening at times and altogether amazing and cried at every delivery.

I loved, dealing with, for the most part, healthy women and their babies. The studying was hard going and the exams terrifying. I was so exhausted when I got home that I would fall asleep and the boys would have to wake me up to make dinner.

Part of the role of the midwife is teaching and this was a real challenge to me as I had never formally taught anyone before. Whoever would have thought I'd be a midwifery tutor one day? Parent craft was the formal type teaching but I found that a lot of new mums needed a lot of support and teaching to look after their new babies so question and answer times were long. One of the questions I was asked at many parent craft sessions was how to test the baby's bathwater, the usual answer was to dip your elbow into the water and if it was warm then it was OK, BUT was the next question, how do you know how warm your elbow is? Common sense isn't so common!!

Home deliveries

My first home delivery was as a student midwife, it happened at night, of course. My midwife mentor called me to say that the lady was in labour and that I should go to the house straight away. This was the lady's second baby and we had looked after her all through her pregnancy so we were all quite comfortable with each other. I arrived before my mentor and did all the necessary things, such as listening to the baby's heart (with an obstetric trumpet, we didn't have electronic Sonic aides then), I palpated her tummy to find the position of the baby and I examined her internally to find out how far her cervix was dilated. The mother was very calm and coping well with her labour and she progressed steadily. The only pain relief she wanted was gas and air with which she coped really well.

All went well, the three year old was playing in the corner of the room and kept reassuring his Mum that she was fine but when she was nearly at the end and shouted a bit he told her that if she didn't behave that she would have to go to the hospital!!! Fortunately she didn't have to go and the baby arrived with the three year old jumping up and down at the end of the bed shouting 'Push Mummy, I can see it coming'. We were all delighted with the baby and finished off with a nice cup of tea.

After eighteen months we all passed our final exams and were delighted to be qualified midwives. I stayed at Worcester for six months and then moved to Bromsgrove (back to my old stomping ground) but this time on the maternity unit. I worked in all areas including ante natal, post natal, antenatal clinic and the delivery suite. It was a busy unit and kept us on the run. At that time we were still giving enemas and shaving women when they were admitted which wasn't nice but was considered the thing to do to ensure a nice clean delivery. Looking back it was almost barbaric but is no longer considered necessary, thank goodness.

One of my patients was a 15 year old whose father locked her in her bedroom to avoid the shame of her being an unmarried mother, her 14 year old boyfriend used to play with a ball outside the clinic while she had her antenatal checks. They split up because she became very irritated with him because he was such a child! She had a good pregnancy and her father came around after discussions with the various help agencies

I saw her through her pregnancy and was at the delivery which she coped with really well. The baby was called Elizabeth, after me.

After six months I moved to community midwifery, mostly in Redditch but I did Bromsgrove cover too. Redditch was a bit rough in parts (mostly the parts I covered!) where you tried to get a boy to watch your car if called out at night and insisted that someone met you at the car to escort you to the house.

There was the woman who wouldn't move from the house until I got there. I was 20 minutes away but she insisted that they wait for me. The ambulance crew sat with her and encouraged her through the last of her labour and I was just in time to catch the baby.

BBAs (Baby Born Away) are babies that deliver at home without a midwife present, this can be because the labour is very quick (as in mothers who have had previous deliveries) or because the woman wanted a home delivery and was advised not to for medical or social reasons and she simply stayed at home and didn't call until it was too late to move her or the baby was born. Sometimes babies are born in the ambulance or the car on the way to the hospital. We even had one born in the car park on a chilly night.

Most midwives could double as contortionists!

The area that I covered had a great variety of homes, from the really upmarket to the worst of the worst. Most people appreciate the upmarket ones but it is difficult for people to understand the really bad ones such as the ones with the brown walls and ceilings caused by the accumulation of nicotine, where the curtains are also brown and permanently closed and all the furniture is sticky with dirt.

The ones where you don't sit down as there is nowhere clean to sit and you always carry a newspaper to put your bag on so that it stays as clean as possible. In these houses you would let the person open doors for you as the door handles were sticky with dirt.

The one where the teenage mother lived with her father and brother, the father was always under a blanket on the settee when I called and masturbated constantly. The brother liked lighting fires in his bed room and the baby became progressively dirtier as time went on. It is difficult to imagine these situations if you haven't been there but I assure you, they are there and all you can do is advise them and contact the much maligned social services who do all they can to help.

Then there was the house where there was a dog poo in the middle of the sitting room floor, The woman said 'Oh ,look what the dogs done', but the turd had a fur coat on it and it had obviously been there for a long time. I suggested that she remove it before I came again.

You can talk your head off and give advice as gently or as forcefully as you can but for some there is no amount of advice will help and then you can only let the health visitors and social workers know about them with a view to what help is available and what they'll accept.

At my antenatal clinic on one of the poorer estates I found that if the women didn't turn up for their appointment I would go to the house to see if there was a problem, this was usually if it was raining but there was rarely a problem and they'd always have the kettle on and say that they knew I wouldn't mind coming to see them at home!!

Then there was the house where they smoked pot and had the most relaxed Alsatian dog and the quietest parrot ever. I was always asked if I would like to join them and although I didn't, there's a lot to be said for secondary smoking. I always left that house feeling at peace with the world!

Both mother and daughter were pregnant and both partners were in prison, if they needed milk for a cup of tea they'd send the three year old out to steal a bottle from a neighbour's doorstep.

There was an ESN (now called special needs) couple, he was 18years old and she was 16years old, they lived in a flat together and insisted on a home birth against all advice. My colleagues and I spent so much time with them during the pregnancy but Peter was terrified of hospitals as his mother had gone into hospital and never came out, no amount of persuasion could make him see that this was a totally different situation to that of his mother dying of cancer.

Ellie wouldn't do anything Peter didn't want her to do so we had to manage as best we could.

Murphy's' law decreed that I should be the one on call the night she went into labour; I alerted everyone that I needed to including ambulance control, the GP on call, the hospital and the other midwife on call and set out. Peter met me at the car park and took me to the house where he proudly showed me a bath half full of water which he had filled by boiling the kettle time after time as he knew that when a baby came you needed lots of hot water. The fact that the bath was filthy and the water less than clean meant nothing to him. Ellie was screaming every time she had a contraction and when she screamed he shouted 'Help her, help her'. I chatted to her about her pains and how often they were coming, I felt her tummy and listened to the baby's heart and that was all fine but when I wanted to examine her internally she screamed, he screamed and said that if I did that he would never touch her again and for emphasis, punched a hole in the wall. I spent hours talking them through all the possibilities and wanted to give her pain relief but he said no. Over the course of the night, cups were thrown, plates were smashed and the threat of violence was always there Peter was like a rumbling volcano, very scary.

The other midwife on call came to support me but went off into the lounge and went to sleep, GREAT!!

After a long hard night of getting nowhere and becoming anxious about the poor exhausted girl I phoned the GP on call who knew both the couple and me. When he arrived I explained the situation and he took the boy aside and talked to him. A few minutes later Peter came out of the kitchen and said that he'd decided that Ellie should go into hospital. The GP and I just smiled and agreed. Ellie had a caesarean section that morning and he insisted on taking her home the next day. All the help they needed was available but was not well received.

In Bromsgrove there was the house where the dog had had a litter of puppies under the sideboard in the bedroom. A really happy family, who all wanted to be there for the birth. The bed was a mattress on the floor; it was a really nice relaxed labour and delivery with much laughter as we tried to keep the puppies off the bed!! That was a very happy night.

One of the houses that I visited was particularly scary for me as the husband had a huge snake that he let loose around the house and was reluctant to put it in its tank while I was there. I had visions of the baby being swallowed whole even though he assured me that that couldn't happen.

Then there was the girl who had been seeing her GP to try to lose weight and then gave birth to a healthy baby in the bathroom at home one night. Her brother woke her Mum and said 'Mum our sis has had a baby in the bathroom'. He was told to go back to bed, it was only a nightmare.

I was the midwife on call that night and went out to check them both over and to transport them both to the hospital, (they were both fine). The whole family were in shock but they rallied quickly and gave her all the support she needed.

Note in her GPs notes – Sudden weight loss, 7lb boy!!

Another woman that I looked after in the community was called Annabel and she wanted a home delivery for her second baby but as there had been problems with her first delivery she was advised against home delivery. It was discussed with her and the risks explained, she was counselled both by her GP and by the Supervisor of midwives all to no avail, Annabel wanted a home delivery and that was that.

The pregnancy went well and all was prepared for the delivery. Annabel called me when she went into labour and I called my supervisor who was acting as second midwife. I also informed ambulance control to warn them in case of emergency.

Annabel's labour was well advanced when I arrived and she had prepared the sitting room by putting down plastic sheeting to protect the carpet and furniture. The toddler was asleep in bed and her husband was away on business.

The labour progressed well and in a short time she delivered a healthy baby boy who weighed seven and a half pounds. When the placenta was delivered I put it in a bowl in the downstairs bathroom to be checked to make sure it was complete later. Then I went back to tidy mum and baby and make them comfortable. All was well and my colleague and I sighed a big sigh of relief. Deliveries are only normal in retrospect and we must always be alert in case of problems arising. Annabel didn't actually say 'I told you so' but it was there, believe me. Unfortunately when I went to check the placenta the dog had eaten it!!!!!!!!!!

Having settled everyone I went home and was back again the next morning at eight o'clock to find Annabel up, dressed, full make up on, baby bathed dressed and fed house cleaned and the toddler still asleep in bed. What organisation.

When I was on call the ambulance control would ring me for a call out and ask was I awake, tell me to sit up and put my glasses on and when I confirmed that I had he would then give me the message. A nice friendly way to do it, now mobile phones tend to cut out the middle man. This is a shame as communication between services is important as it keeps the personal element alive.

I loved my time on the community and made many friends both clients and students. I even delivered one of my students two children.

There seems to be some confusion about midwifery as to what we actually do and I am frequently asked, after working a shift, 'how many babies have you delivered today?' as if we just stand there and catch them as they fly out. Midwifery is so all inclusive of life and families and caring that, unless you've been there it's difficult to understand, for a short period of time we become a part of that family and it's wonderful.

I have been called many things –

The doctor lady.

The nurse

The lady with the baby in her bag.

The madwife.

The midwife.

That bl----dy nuisance.

But best of all, from a four year old who looked through the letter box and called to his Mummy, It's the baby catcher.

Continuing Education

Having worked for a few years as a midwife I moved back into the maternity unit and I had the opportunity to do the ENB998 course which was, Teaching and Assessing in Clinical Practice. I really enjoyed the course and put it to good use back on the ward. I enjoyed using my newfound skills and was surprised at how well it was received.

My boys were growing fast and I was always on the go, I was Mums taxi service, homework helper and all the other things that Mums do without thinking. Life was great, if a little tiring.

The ENB998 course led to me applying for and being accepted for the Advanced Diploma in Midwifery Course and ultimately to a degree in midwifery education, an Honours degree course which I did at Wolverhampton University. Although my mother-in-law thought that I was too old for 'all this studying'.

Even the interview to get on to the ADM was hard and I didn't think I'd make it but I did even though it stretched my brain in all directions!! So much to study, so much more to learn and so much more writing of essays and projects.

One of the nurse tutors at the hospital that had seconded me told me that I was addicted to learning. I think it was meant to be a put down but he was close to the truth.

My first published article, Positions in Labour, was a project that I did for the ADM. It was published in the Nursing Times. For some reason the tutor didn't believe that I'd written it. Why don't people take me seriously? I was very proud of that article and have even had students quote it in their own essays.

Some of the students that did the ADM then went on to study the PGCE(Post Graduate Certificate in Education) I wasn't sure that I wanted to go into full time teaching so didn't apply. Then I had a letter through the post offering me the chance to do a degree in education the following year. To fill in the time I did a Gateway Course at the local college which included 'A' level biology, sociology and general studies. As usual I was the oldest student!! Some of us are just late starters.

Degree in education at Wolverhampton

I had never seen myself as university material but thank goodness someone at the interviews did. I had a lot of support from family and friends, especially the boys who were now 21 and 17 years old.

There were 16 of us on the course and I was the oldest AGAIN. We were all very nervous and each of us, it turned out was very unsure of ourselves and expected to be ousted when they found out that we weren't as bright as they thought but eventually we discovered that we were quite bright and could actually do this teaching thing. I took a while!!

It was a sharp learning curve over the next 18 months and really hard work. So much to learn, so much to do, so many essays, lesson planning, teaching practice, lectures. So many new ideas to take on board and gadgets to understand. So many new people to liaise with.

And at the same time my marriage was falling apart.

What a short sentence to cover such devastation.

My marriage split up in 1992 and it came as a complete surprise, although in retrospect, it didn't surprise me at all. They say that everything is clear in retrospect and this was certainly true for me. I spent 2 years in denial.

Many things were going on in our lives at the time; I was on the way up having completed two courses and was in the middle of a degree course when the split came. David, on the other hand had been made redundant, had started his own company which had gone to the wall and he was now unemployed. Robert, our younger son, at 17years was being troublesome, to say the least; also our older son had gone to live in Holland and I missed him terribly, so there were many factors contributing to our stress levels.

During the two years leading up to the split I was constantly making excuses for David's behaviour and moodiness, his lack of self-esteem and general attitude. I made all the compromises and dealt with a lot of Roberts 'rubbish' so David didn't have to deal with that as well.

I thought I was being a good wife and mother. Marc leaving home was a great loss to me as I saw him as my hold on normality, as he was easy to live with, good humoured (most of the time) and had a sense of humour which seemed to have disappeared from David's life. Marc left in the June and we celebrated David's mother's birthday the same month and in the August he left and my life was in tatters. During the time before the split I wrote –

The sadness of Love

You are still here but I feel bereaved

I hold you but you're not there

We talk but you don't speak

We live around each other with no point of
contact

We're not even good friends anymore

You live here but keep your heart hidden from
me

I don't know how to repair the rift

And you don't seem to want to

We used to laugh, to touch and to make love

But it's all going. Not quite gone

But twenty years of life slowly trickling away

And I can't catch it

As it slips through the net of your indifference.

However life, as they say, must go on and so I completed my degree and was given a contract to teach by the University of Central England.

Teaching at University of Central England

Midwifery teaching for the University of Central England was generally carried out at Sorrento hospital in Moseley, Birmingham or at Good Hope hospital in Sutton Coldfield. The school at Sorrento was an old house and at Good Hope, a purpose built school. The contrast was amazing and each had a very distinctive atmosphere.

Teaching at Sorrento

Conversion students were students who were converting from enrolled nurse to general nursing and came to us to do their obstetric placement which lasted four weeks and they always complained that it wasn't enough. They were so eager and enthusiastic and were delighted to be involved in anything that they were given the chance to do. They were a real pleasure to teach. I was their nominated tutor and organised their teaching, lesson planning, placements and assessment. I loved it.

The frightening students for me were the midwifery students, probably because I felt that they knew almost as much as me. It turned out that they didn't but when you're doing teaching practice you don't realise that. A big boost for me was when I asked the students to critique my lessons and received some great feedback, I was astonished but delighted.

My mentor, Thelma Bamfield was lovely and I felt very safe with her until she made me teach on my own....PANIC but she sat in on the sessions, looked over my teaching plans and generally supported me all along the way.

The first time I went to the college I asked for her and was told to follow the stink of Galois, which I did and found her tucked away in a little office at the back of the building where we spent many hours together, happy hours, agonising hours, weeping hours and she lent me her shoulder to cry on when my husband left me.

I was so lucky really that I had so much support when David left, otherwise I might not have made it. Actually I would have because I wouldn't give him the satisfaction of seeing me fail. As it happened I didn't fail I passed and was given a contract to teach at the University of Central England.

As my older son had left home and was living in Holland, my husband had left home and my younger son who had been really strong for me was thinking about moving out so I decided to broaden my life and horizons and applied to join Voluntary Service Overseas

In 1992 my decree absolute came through and I went to train midwives in the Maldives

My book Maldives Musings is the story of my two years in the Maldives where I went to train foolhumas, the local birth attendants but when I arrived I was told that they had enough of those and could I write a six month midwifery course? Well, what do you say when you're so far from home? I agreed and set about writing, teaching both classroom and practical work, I had to liaise with both the college and the hospital and have my scheme of work approved by both the President's office and the University of Bangalore in India.

It was a great challenge for me, the students were already the equivalent of our SENs and were desperate to learn, they absorbed everything I threw at them and were lovely.

I can't say that I enjoyed every minute of the two years but it gave me back my life and confidence and I found that I liked myself again.

I should tell you that the word foolhumas translates as 'Mother of the belly button'. Sweet, eh?

Back to the UK

When I came back to the UK after spending 2 years in the Maldives, I moved back into the family home and I hated it, it was totally alien without the family there. I have always said that it is a mistake to go back and I was right.

All my old friends were there and welcomed me with open arms and expected me to fit right back in, doing the same things together as we had done before I left. I felt that they had remained static whereas I had moved on. I felt that their lives were shallow and mine was much broader. I'm not saying that I thought myself better than them but that I had changed and they hadn't.

How arrogant was that?

I found it difficult to come to terms with the differences between the Maldives way of life and the way of life back here where the biggest problem people seemed to have been when their next holiday would be as opposed to the relatively basic way of life in the Maldives.

It was a joy to sleep in a proper house again as I had spent the last two years living in a breeze block house with a tin roof, a separate kitchen, complete with resident rat and doing my washing in a red plastic bucket. I soon learned to live with all this luxury back home!! It was heaven being able to buy what I wanted as far as food was concerned but for some strange reason I had to have a tin of tuna in my cupboard at all times. Something to do with living on tuna for two years!! I never opened it but felt happy with it there.

I sold the house and moved into a two bedroom flat in the same town and gradually settled down a bit.

Whilst I was away I had become a grandmother for the first time and now there was another one on the way. It was lovely to see my family and catch up on all the news but I missed Colin, he and I had met in the Maldives, he was a water and sanitation engineer and we got on really well. Colin stayed on an extra year and when he came back he moved in with me. All was well for a while, I was teaching at Worcester College, part time and also part time at Leicester University. In between I worked at the hospital where I had worked previously, again part time. I also helped with preparing (VSO) volunteers who were going out to teach and interviewed prospective student midwives at Worcester College, one of whom told me that she felt that she would make a good midwife because she was an actress and had played a nurse on the stage!!! When asked how she would cope with the occasional tragedies that happen in midwifery she replied that she would keep a stiff upper lip and not let the woman see that she was upset. WRONG. This girl was not accepted and was most put out and demanded to know why. Hmmmmm, I wonder.

So I was busy, busy and Colin became more and more frustrated with his life as he felt useless and so he returned to VSO and went off to South Africa.

Our relationship survived the Maldives and although we remained good friends it couldn't survive anywhere else. This happens quite a lot where couples are thrown together in an alien situation but it only works in that time and that place, it doesn't work anywhere else. It's called propinquity.

By this time I had had enough of teaching; I enjoyed it but missed the patient contact. It was actually not the teaching I had had enough of, it was all of the other elements involved in teaching, the lesson planning, the assessing, the marking, the invigilating and last but not least the politics!!

So, here I was, no ties, looking for something to do to move on, and up popped an advert in the media for midwives in Gibraltar. YES!!!!!!!

Geography and history of Gibraltar

Gibraltar is a peninsula that hangs on the end of Spain, it is the southernmost tip of Europe, it is about three miles square and has a population of around 30,0000 residents, this number fluctuates with the season and the influx of visitors from Spain and the cruise liners that call into Gibraltar. Most of the residents live in the main town area which is like an ants nest, busy on many levels (mostly up!!) There are also lots of blocks of apartments built on reclaimed land and another residential area around the other side of the rock called Catalan Bay. The people of Catalan Bay see themselves as different (better than) the people from the town but can't say how.

Gibraltar has been a British Protectorate since it was ceded to the British in 1713 and its people are fiercely loyal to the Queen and all things British although Spain claims sovereignty, a referendum in 2008 proved that Gibraltarians want to remain British.

Gibraltar has a rich history and many sites of interest but sadly the visitors mainly see the shops in the main street and go on the Rock Tour which visits some of the places of interests but doesn't do the place justice. It would appear that all visitors are interested in are the apes and tax free cigarettes and booze. Perhaps this is a little harsh as their time in port is limited.

Moving to Gibraltar

I was interviewed in London in the November 1998 and then had a long wait to find out if I had been successful. Finally in the New Year I was informed that I had been successful and was due to start in March 1999.

I left England expecting good weather when we landed but no, it was raining. The landing was pretty awful as it was windy and raining and as the plane came into Gibraltar it was very bumpy and everyone was screaming. I assumed that they were all locals and were just messing about but when we actually landed and everyone started clapping and cheering it hit me that it had actually been very dangerous. I learned later that Gibraltar is one of the five most dangerous airstrips in the world!!!!!!!

There were four of us on the plane who were taking up midwifery posts at the hospital. Well, actually there was more than four as Hazel came with her partner, Rebecca came with her sister and Jenny came with her husband, son and daughter, so a grand total of nine. A reception committee was at the airport to welcome us and to take us to our accommodation.

Before I went to Gibraltar, my sisters had been on holiday in Benalmadena which is just up the coast from Gibraltar and they had brought me back a local paper from Gibraltar having been on a day trip to 'sus' the place out for me and to my horror I was going to be living in a high rise flat. Little did I realise that much of Gibraltar is high rise, of necessity, as land is so limited.

At the airport we were handed over to our mentors and were taken to our new places. I was given to Flordeliz (a Gibraltarian midwife) who took me to my flat in Watergardens. I was delighted with it, so bright and airy, four floors up with a view of the marina and a balcony on two sides, high rise wasn't so bad after all.

There was a basic food parcel and all amenities were on. I had sheets, pillow cases, pillows and towels but no duvet and it was cold, I wasn't expecting cold or rain and said as much to Flordeliz who pointed out that it was still winter and that the rain was needed.

The next morning after a cold night when I slept with my coat on the bed I went shopping for a duvet and a hot water bottle. On my way back to the flat I tripped over and was picked up by three little old ladies who brushed me down and sent me on my way with the beginnings of a black eye!! A good start!

The next day we had to find the personnel office (now known as Human Resources, of course). It was pouring with rain and I met up with Jenny and her family (so nice to see a familiar face) also looking for the office which we finally found in another street from the hospital where we turned up looking like drowned rats. Contracts were signed and we then went to the maternity unit to collect uniforms and off duty times and to have a look around.

The building was old but felt warm and friendly (little did I know!), there were two delivery rooms, an admission room a special care baby unit, a nursery, two side rooms and an eight bedded ward, a much smaller unit than any of us was used to. There was also a day room with a fantastic view of Gibraltar and the bay.

There was a huge culture shock for both the Gibraltarians and for us. The local nurses and midwives didn't want us there and were very defensive. We came in with UK ideas about how things should be done. We stuck to the rules and so were considered 'antipatica' or unsympathetic especially by the visiting relatives.

Other things that set us apart:-

We didn't spread the word about deliveries to the rest of Gibraltar but let the families do that, whereas previously whoever could get to the phone first would let all their friends know the outcome of a delivery, which meant that sometimes the whole of Gibraltar knew before the extended family did.

We didn't understand that it was common practice for ALL the staff to attend a delivery and I was in trouble one night when I asked some of them to leave the room as it felt like New Street Station, they went to the night sister's office and threatened to walk out. **I learned.**

We weren't used to the whole family sitting outside the maternity unit awaiting the birth from the onset of labour, waiting all night in the draughty corridor, even in the winter time. Nor were we used to the whole family being allowed in to see the new baby as soon as possible after delivery, I quite like that and even now it still happens although we have a new hospital and a nice warm waiting room, the family and friends are allowed in to see the baby before the mother even has a chance to shower and change.

It was also a sign of a busy ward if there were relatives waiting outside when we came on duty.

Patients going for caesarean sections were no exception to the family rule and everyone was there from the time they were admitted to the time they returned from theatre. It was a nightmare, the baby was taken from the theatre to the ward by the midwife who had to run the gauntlet of the family who were waiting outside theatre and insisted on having a look at the baby and giving it a kiss before the midwife could escape down the stairs to the ward with the baby still wrapped in its blanket.

We were used to total patient care which meant that we looked after both mother and baby whereas in this maternity unit the nursery nurses looked after the baby and the midwives looked after the mother. Not ideal but it had its good points.

We were used to ordering stock as and when we needed it but here we had to return empties before more was supplied. This extended even to syringes which were supplied on a one for one basis.

Central Sterile Supply Department (CSSD) was very limited and the maternity unit had its own steriliser for forceps and small articles and lo and behold, I found myself using Cheatles forceps again after forty years. Talk about back to basics.

However, we tried very hard not to say 'in the UK', too often as you could see the hackles rise but it was difficult at times.

The ward routine was very civilised, we arrived at eight and had the report in the office, the babies were put into the nursery and the patients had their breakfast in the day room whilst the cleaners cleaned the ward. By ten thirty all post natal checks were done, babies bathed and returned to their mothers who were then served coffee.

It was then time for us to sit in the office and have our coffee, usually with sister and whichever consultant was on duty. As the newspaper was delivered to the ward we were also expected to help with the crossword puzzle.

On Sunday mornings the nurses would make a cooked breakfast for all the staff with all the trimmings.

Obviously this all depended on what was happening on the ward, labourers, admissions and etc. but usually we had coffee together.

The patients were well cared for and we spent a lot of time with each of them as there were no parent craft sessions for expectant women. They had a lot of help from the extended family but as many of the ideas were a little odd we found that although they liked the idea of parent craft, they still wanted the family input. It was little things like putting a small piece of cotton wool on the baby's forehead to stop the baby's hiccups, strangely it seemed to work.

Another thing that was totally alien to us was the fact that the mothers expected baby girls to have their ears pierced before they went home, (most of them) and the midwife was expected to do this. We were horrified but soon learned to do it. It was surprisingly easy with very little reaction from the baby and rarely any blood. I believe it started at the request of the, then, paediatrician as it was previously being done by many and various people with little or no experience and questionable methods and hygiene which led to babies with infected ear lobes. He considered it to be a better idea if midwives were trained to do it and in all my time here I have never seen a baby with an infected ear lobe.

However, this practice was stopped by a management group who came from the UK to review our practices and were totally shocked at this 'barbaric practice'. Now the women have the baby's ears pierced at the pharmacy or the tattoo parlour at a significant cost.

Ear piercing is a good way of telling the girls from the boys as my son and his partner found out when they came to visit me and people kept referring to my granddaughter who at eight months had very little hair, as 'he'. She's now 13 and has her ears pierced.

Night Duty

Night duty was interesting, there were the permanent night staff and one of us 'antipaticas'! The patients were, generally, settled down by 10.30 and the lights turned out. Then the desk in the office was cleared and laid with a clean sheet and food put out for all to share, although the food from the kitchen was excellent and freshly cooked most staff took their own. Once the meal was finished the desk was cleared again and out came the Scrabble which went on late into the night and causing niggles and arguments about what was and was not allowed. The Scrabble book was consulted regularly!!!

Night duty brings with it a sort of madness at times, like when we were going to check on the patients, one of the nursing assistants would get out her imaginary motorbike and rev it up and I'd pretend to get on the back and hold on and we would go zooming into the ward to make sure the women and babies were OK. Seeing this in writing it looks as though we were complete loonies but night duty gets you that way at times. Sometimes we would be dancing on the desk at 4am and singing silly songs but we were actually very responsible, most of the time.

We would all take something to do to pass the time and one of the nurses decided that she wanted to make a stained glass window to go over her front door so we designed it, she brought in the glass and we made it. It turned out really well; she tells me that it's still there and looking good.

Of course, at night the cockroaches came out and they were BIG. We found them in the kitchen, on the stairs, in the bathroom and even in the baby's cots at times. Horrible. I may have mentioned it before but I hate cockroaches. On day duty you always knew they were there but you didn't see them. At night they were highly visible, ugh!!!!

There was also a rat run outside the ward and we would often see the rats trotting around. Why do rats always look as if they're on a mission?

Afternoons were generally quiet, the women sleeping after their lunch to rev up for the onslaught of the visitors whom Agnes, a nursery nurse, kept under strict control, two to a bed and no more. She actually sat at the door with her crocheting, marking them in and out.

Meantime we sat in the office knitting, sewing or just chatting, again, very civilised and definitely not what we were used to. Sometimes we would join the women in the dayroom after visiting time and either chat or there was often a jigsaw on the go, although the visiting children had helped a little at times! The ward sister was one of the 'old school' who held court and regaled us with stories about how things used to be; she was a great raconteur and kept us amused. This is not to say that she was any less efficient and in control, she was always well aware of everything that went on in the unit and beyond.

There was an organised feel to the place and the women got the best of care. So organised, in fact that our first weekend on duty we were left in charge, talk about feeling our way. The midwifery part was not a problem but we had no idea who to contact if there was a problem but there again we were midwives so we coped!! We were also back to split shifts again.

Christmas was a nice time, the ward was decorated, food and drinks were put in the sideward for the staff and as in days of old the consultant came to carve the turkey for staff and patients, a lovely traditional Christmas day. We also had a visit from the Governor and the First Minister and all of the families of the patients were welcome all day.

Around Christmas time there were parties in an empty ward downstairs and everyone brought food, there was music and all wards and departments were invited. One of the delicacies was Henrys balls. Henry was the Danish husband of one of the nurses and he made his meat balls every year, they were really good. Sadly Henry has died so no more meat balls.

There was also a Christmas dinner for all of the staff at the Casino Ballroom, a noisy, chatty, singing, dancing night that everyone enjoyed. It was lovely to get dressed up and be looked after, even if only for one night. There were even presents for all of us from the ward sister, a small token but much appreciated.

One of the most touching things for me in Gibraltar was that there were often thank you notices in the local paper, to the midwife who had delivered the baby, how sweet. Not only that, but there were often small personal gifts, not to mention the cakes and chocolates that were sent to the ward for us. Gibraltarians are very generous people.

My first delivery was a neighbour who was totally shocked when I asked her if she was alright with me looking after her as we lived so near to each other, I don't think that she realised that she had a choice and said that she was happy to have me. I looked after her with her second child as well and still see her around the town.

I think that one of the main problems for me in moving to Gibraltar was the fact that everyone spoke English and therefore I expected them to think like we did. This was not so, Gibraltar has its' own culture and way of thinking and DEFINITELY NOT like the English although they are more British than the British in some ways. Gibraltar has all the same bank holidays as England and also celebrates the Queen's birthday and Commonwealth day.

They also have their own language which is a mixture of Spanish and English which is called Janito and this was much employed when we first arrived, probably to keep us in our place as outsiders and also to highlight our differences. There was great resentment and resistance on the part of the Gibraltarian nurses and midwives, which was difficult to deal with at times as we didn't know what we were doing wrong.

Gibraltar is like a small village where everybody knows everybody else and they all know everybody's business, this can lead you to one of the two following feelings,

1. How lovely to feel that everyone knows me and I feel so safe.

2. How awful that everybody knows me and my business.

These feelings can vary from day to day and can lead to feelings of terrible claustrophobia and discontent and it wasn't long before I started looking at houses in Spain and found just what I wanted in a village called Guadiaro,

20 minutes over the border and within easy commuting distance.

The Babe

Came into my life when she was 10 months old and has sat in my heart ever since. She was taken to the cats' refuge because her previous owners' son became allergic to her at about the same time as they had new furniture!!! She is black and white and was full of life, especially in the middle of the night, as is the way with cats. When I bought my house in Spain she and I would go there on my days off, she loved the freedom of the three floored house and the terrace and would dash about like a mad thing. At 14 years, she still dashes about but not so much, probably something to do with falling out of the third floor bedroom window twice and from the fourth floor terrace once and landing on concrete!! She has used up most of her nine lives now.

Community service

The idea was for the four of us to set up a community midwifery service in Gibraltar to include home bookings, post natal care and to set up parent craft sessions, none of which had been available to the women before.

Rebecca and I were sent out to buy bags in which to carry our necessities and found just the right ones. We were also sent to buy a small fridge for the drugs that needed to be stored at low temperature as prior to our coming they had been stored in the kitchen fridge which was far from ideal.

The expectation was that we would set up and run the community service which we did very successfully. All of our visits were done on foot (well, mostly) as some places were difficult to get to and there was very little parking in the town. Anyone who knows me knows that I don't do walking and would drive around until I found parking, this led to a few parking tickets!!!!

Hospital antenatal Clinics

Ante natal clinics were insane, there was no appointment system and all the women turned up at 1.30pm, hoping to be seen early. The clinic waiting area was a short corridor and was always choc a bloc with women, children, shopping, push chairs and general mayhem. Despite this it was a happy gathering place and everyone took their turn. In the summer there were usually less people as they would be down on the beach. We often thought about running the clinic on the beach itself!!

Bookings

This is the first meeting with the midwife and when all the personal details are recorded. Until now it had always been done in the clinic and it was a great novelty for us to visit the women at home and I know that some of them thought that we were spying on them rather than giving them more privacy but they got used to it and appreciated the service.

Uniforms

During our first year our uniforms changed three times. First we were given winter uniforms, blue dress with long sleeves and then, white summer dresses with short sleeves and finally blue dresses with short sleeves. We didn't wear caps but were expected to wear a belt. I hadn't worn a belt for years and worried that mine wouldn't reach around my waist but it did and it was nice to wear my buckle again. This didn't last, of course and we were soon dressed in blue pyjamas which were by far the best and most comfortable of uniforms which are still worn today.

Another part of my work was teaching student nurses who were doing the maternity module of their training, I taught the anatomy and physiology aspect and another midwife covered ethics. Other than that the students were taught by the tutors in the school of nursing.

As well as the ward upstairs there was also a six bedded ward downstairs which was used when we had more patients. At times it was used for overflow from the medical wards which meant that we had patients with chronic problems that just needed basic care. These were mostly little old ladies who were delighted to be with us and to see the babies when they went up to the dayroom for meals. The mothers were pleased to see them as well, except for the table manners of these old dears which left much to be desired!!! There was even a time when we had old men too but these weren't easily pleased and it only happened once.

Within a year of our arrival another great change shook the maternity unit........... **male midwives**!!!!!! There have been a few over the years since then but it is Miguel, the first one that has stayed with us. We weren't sure how the women would react to male midwives but there have been very few who were concerned and the men are well accepted as a rule.

Another interesting thing that happened was that Jenny and I were interviewed by a television film crew who were talking to expats up and down the coast, in various occupations, to see how they were getting along with their new lives in the sun. I believe the program went out on midlands television but we didn't see it and we weren't mobbed in the streets as TV stars!!

I cannot leave the old hospital without mentioning a few of the characters that inhabited the place and left their mark.

There was the self-confessed Scottish bitch and yes, she really was and heaven help you if she didn't like you. I was lucky as neither of us suffered fools gladly and we got along... mostly!! Some of the younger staff were upset by her at times.

There was Pepito who was the messenger 'boy' who was 40 if he was a day, always cheerful, and always smiling. He's still there, still smiling.

There was Rose, one of the nurses who was a great worker but a bit of a rebel who gave lots of advice to the patients that may have been a bit dodgy and who smoked in the ward bathroom and sang all day, songs from the 60's, she knew all the words.

Then there was the midwife who cried and kicked the filing cabinets if she didn't get the off duty that she wanted. Very grown up!!!

One of the midwives considered our ordering of what we referred to as a Chinky takeaway meal, to be racist! She also hated us to refer to the women we were looking after as 'My lady'. Strange person!

Everywhere has its' characters and they're great, they make life interesting.

Rescued

When I had been in Gibraltar for around 8 months I developed gall stones which if you have had them you'll know that the pain is excruciating. I was very fortunate in that they were diagnosed and dealt with very promptly and I was sent to London to have them removed.

On my return to Gibraltar I was off sick for a couple of weeks so decided to make use of the time to refurbish an old armchair that I had acquired. This required the removal of the old paint on the arms and legs and to this end I had put the chair out on my balcony to apply the paint remover.

While I was doing this the Babe came to see what I was doing and to prevent her from harm I gave the balcony door a little nudge so that she couldn't get out. HUH, I immediately realised my mistake as the door clicked shut marooning me on the balcony!!!!!! So here I was 4 floors up, stuck, without a hope of getting in.

Whenever I had sat outside before there had been people around, not this time. I waited and waited, getting a bit chilly now, and then I saw a colleague walking her dog and shouted to her, she waved back and carried on, so I shouted louder and she realised that I needed help. She came up to the mezzanine level which was one floor below my balcony and passed me up a blanket on a broomstick and said that she had called the fire brigade.

Well, the fire engine came with all sirens blaring, very embarrassing. What they did, was remove the double glazing from the bedroom window so that they could get in and open the door for me. They then spent an hour reassembling the window. Bless them, they were so kind. The next morning on the daily police report it was reported that the fire brigade had rescued a woman from a balcony in Watergardens. Fame at last!

Moving to Spain

I bought my house in Spain in October but didn't move in until the following February which gave me time to get set up and shop, shop, shop. I loved getting all the right things for the house which was on a side street and was part of an old cinema. My neighbour over the road tells me that she remembers the film being run by a tractor engine when she was a child. It amazes me that they would build a cinema in such a small village as it was in the 1950's. The village has grown enormously since I moved in in 2000 and the nearest cinema is miles away.

All of my neighbours are Spanish and only two of them speak English but we get along, with my bit of Spanish and their goodwill. I did take lessons but found that I could manage and more often than not I was with English speaking people anyway. I was just lazy really but avoided the English way of **SPEAKING**

SLOWLY AND LOUDLY TO MAKE MYSELF UNDERSTOOD!!

It took a while to get used to the fact that Spanish people are loud and for the first few weeks I thought that they were continually fighting and about to kill each other. Thankfully I soon worked it out but I still find it hard at times and now when I'm in England it seems very quiet.

The New Hospital

In 2006 we moved to the new hospital which was down in the town area as opposed to halfway up the rock. This made it easier for the women getting to clinic and also when they were in labour and I'm sure that the incidence of high blood pressure became less as they didn't have to walk up the hill.

The new hospital was wonderful, all open spaces and small wards, modern delivery suites and all new, up to date equipment. No dark corners where cockroaches could lurk and a proper security system. No need for an Agnes guarding the door at visiting times!

With the move to the new hospital and employing more and younger, enthusiastic midwives the women's choices have increased in that the rooms are bigger allowing for more mobility in labour, there is more equipment such as the large balls to sit on, the armchairs and even a large bath that they can labour in if they wish. No birthing pool as yet but I'm sure that it will come.

They also have a choice of pain relief and can request an epidural which was unheard of in the old place.Things are improving all the time and the service is much appreciated by the women and their families.

Retirement!!!

When I reached 60 I was told that I had to retire as I was employed by the government and that was the rule. A petition was sent to Human Resources and one of the consultants pleaded my case but no, the rules are the rules and off I went after a nice party and speeches and gifts.

For three months I enjoyed my retirement, caught up on years of lost sleep (I began to think that I had sleeping sickness!) caught up on lots of things that needed doing in the house, spent more time with the cats, (by this time Julio my ginger tom had joined us) and generally relaxed.

Then I had a call from the hospital to ask if I would cover a shift and I've been covering shifts ever since, usually only two or three a month but enough to keep me occupied and out of trouble!! It also means that I have to keep up to date with the latest trends and education and reregister with the Nurses and Midwives Council on an annual basis.

Working as a bank (or supply) midwife has many advantages,

o   You can say no if you don't want to work.

o   You can enjoy your work without getting involved in the politics.

o   You can do your shift and go home and forget about it.

o   You don't take your work home.

For me the disadvantage of doing bank work is that I never know when it will be my last delivery or my last shift and this can be a little unsettling as I really love midwifery and will be sad when it comes to an end. I only came for a year and 14 years on I'm still here.

I have met so many people here, made friends here and I even begin to think that I am, almost, accepted by the Gibraltarians, even though I haven't actually been here for the requisite 25 years!!!!!!!

I have delivered many babies and cared for many women, at times it has been a challenge, and sometimes frustrating but always satisfying.

There's something wonderful about babies, the feel of them, and the smell of them (most of the time!), how wonderfully alert they are, the grasp of a tiny hand and the feel of their breath on your face. All of these things I will miss. This year I became an honorary grandma as my friend's son, who I delivered, 22 years ago, has just become a father, how wonderful is that?

I love my life style now, I have time to think and read. I have time for my family and my hobbies of drawing, writing and knitting. I love being a member of the Kings Chapel Singers in Gibraltar where we sing every Tuesday evening and then go to the pub for cheesy chips. I have time to socialise and am become 'A lady who lunches'.

I'm also involved with a group of women with OCD (Obsessive Cat Disorder) who rescue and re home cats, a very worthy bunch they are too but CATS? What about poor children? Don't get me started!!!!!!!!!

End Bit

I started this book with the intention of highlighting the changes and advances in nursing and midwifery care over the years and I hope that I've done that but it has also shown me that some things never change and that can be good as well. It has given me so much pleasure to go back and remember people and places that have brought me to where I am and I hope that you have enjoyed it too.